Running

Everything You Need to Know About Running from Beginner to Expert

James Sinclair

James Sinclair

quote or paraphrase any part or the content within this book without the consent of the author or copyright owner. Legal action will be pursued if this is breached.

Table of Contents

Introduction

Are you looking for a way to reduce weight? Are you not able to make up your mind as to what to do to reduce weight? You don't have to worry anymore. We are here with the answer: Running. Yes, running. It is one of the most popular and healthiest ways to reduce weight without stressing your body out too much.

In this book, we bring to you some knowledge packed chapters that will be your guide to losing weight by running and a healthy diet to go along with it.

So without any further ado, let us get started. I want to thank you for choosing this book and I hope that you find the content informative and helpful in your weight loss journey.

James Sinclair

Chapter 1

YOU WERE BORN TO RUN!

"Runners are the ultimate celebration people. Running is just so intense, you're really experiencing life to the fullest." – Bill Rodgers

Make no mistake about it, the so-called "runners' high" is not just an imaginary one...it's real. It's one of the best reasons to believe that humans like, well, you and me, were born to run.

One of my favorite books in the world is *Born to Run* by Christopher McDougall. It's the book that really changed my life, in particular my running life. Aside from the very inspiring story of a great runner named El Caballo Blanco and the native Mexican running tribe called Tarahumaras (who run ultra-marathon distances for leisure on nothing but make shift sandals), it also enumerates several reasons why we humans were born to run. Knowing these reasons encouraged me to continue and achieve milestones in my own running journey, which at that time was on a plateau.

Knowing that we were born to run encouraged – nay, compelled me because I now have no reason to quit or stop running – me to continue running and make great strides in it. As such, I dedicate the very first chapter of this book to enumerating and explaining to you why you were born to run. I believe that knowing these reasons will also encourage you to either take up running or continue doing it.

RUN TO LIVE

"We run when we're scared, we run when we're ecstatic, we run away from our problems and run around for a good time." – Christopher McDougall in his best-selling book *Born to Run*

Running is an excellent way to experience the joys of life and reduce its pain and sorrows. I can attest to that. Whenever I encounter challenges that seem to be too big for me at the moment, I run. Not away from it, mind you but around the village in order to release all my pent up stress energy, which allows me to relax and put my mind in the best possible condition to either solve the problem or figure out the next steps toward it. Often times, nervous tension energy distracts us too much to concentrate on solving a problem and when we run, we release much of that energy to help calm us down and focus.

Another reason why we were born to run is to live. In fact, our primitive ancestors couldn't have survived much if they didn't know how to run. Can you imagine surviving in the wild, where savage beasts abound, simply by brisk walking yourself to safety when pursued by such? Unless those beasts are very poor brisk walkers, your chances of surviving are as high as skinny models' chances of going for seconds on a buffet party.

Aside from surviving ferocious animal attacks, our primitive ancestors also ran in order to hunt for food. Think about this, primitive men weren't born with spears in their hands, right? Given that, how'd you think they hunted for food? Well, they were born with feet, which they used for what is called persistence hunting.

Persistence hunting is a way of hunting animals by tracking them continuously by running and walking until they are exhausted enough to be, you know, hunted. You may be wondering, aren't most animals much faster runners than us humans? You are right in such wondering, my friend. What most people don't know however is that humans are built for endurance running and most animals aren't.

But what made it possible for our ancestors to engage in persistence hunting for survival? One word: sweat!

SWEET SWEAT

Have you ever seen your pet dogs or cats sweat? Have you ever seen horses sweat? Have you ever seen fish sweat? I'd bet your answer is no. This doesn't mean that they don't sweat, save probably for your goldfish. It only means they don't have the ability to sweat as much as we can.

Take for example your pet dog or cat. Their sweating is concentrated primarily on their faces (particularly the nose and mouth) and paws. They don't sweat anywhere else. This is why you notice that their noses and mouths are usually wet, especially on hot days. Horses and cows also don't sweat as much as you do on a hot and humid day. What this means is that their cooling mechanisms aren't anywhere near as efficient as people's and as such, makes them susceptible to overheating and exhaustion much quicker than us – 10 to 15 minutes on average. Because they overheat faster, our ancestors were eventually able to subdue and, yum, eat them.

Have you ever tried taking your dog out for a run, especially on a hot and humid day? Do your dog a favor and just go for a walk with him or her because they won't be able to keep up. Their cooling systems aren't anywhere near yours or mine.

GLYCOGEN

Glyco what? Ok, geek-speak aside, glycogen is the unused glucose (our cells' gasoline if you will) that is stored in our livers for future use. Glucose is what becomes of the carbohydrates we consume. Think of the liver as the body's fuel tank. When you exercise in the morning before eating breakfast, this is the primary fuel your muscles use.

It is believed that most humans' livers contain 20 miles worth of glycogen on average. That's quite a long run, if you ask me. Just like a high-performance sports car relies on a very efficient cooling system and the best fuels to go far and fast, so does the human body. Our bodies' ability to store much more glycogen than most other animals combined with a much better cooling system (sweat) allowed our ancestors to survive via persistence hunting. It also makes us natural born runners.

RUNNERS' ANATOMY

No amount of glycogen stores and cooling system would be enough to make us born to run. What's possibly more important is our physiological structure. Look, snakes have a very efficient cooling system – they're cold-blooded for crying out loud! But do they have the body parts to run? I say no.

What makes us humans stand out from other mammals that run the earth are the spring-like ligaments and tendons in the feet, butt muscles, and our big toe. Let's take a closer look at why these conspire to make us natural born runners.

Tendons and ligaments in our feet help us run efficiently because these parts make it possible for the body to absorb impact and propel the body much like what springs and shock absorbers do. Let's face it, running is an impact activity (i.e., subjects the body to impact when feet hit the pavement). Tendons and ligaments help absorb much of that impact, store the energy produced by it, and release it to propel us forward. To further illustrate the point, have you ever tried running with your foot locked straight? Now you have an idea of the why tendons and ligaments help absorb impact and the resulting energy as well as to release such energy for propulsion.

But wait, there's more! Pardon the pun but yes, our butts are another reason why we're much better runners than animals. To be able to run quite a distance, we also need to stabilize our trunks...and I ain't talkin' about Speedos here. Butt muscles − better known as glutes (short for its scientific name gluteus maximus and minimus) − attach the hip to the base of the spine, making it possible for us to run with great stability. Glutes also make us look good in tucked in pants! Don't believe me? Check out a chimpanzee in pants and see how hip-hoppish that looks!

The big toe is also a big difference maker when it comes to running. Being the last body part to leave the ground when running, it's the main body part used for pushing off the body much like the fingertips are the ultimate follow-through instruments when shooting a basketball. What makes the big toe such a big difference maker is the fact that unlike the big toes of apes and other non-running related species, ours is pretty much lined up with the other toes. In layman's terms, this lined-up position makes for a great running advantage.

KNOWING IS HALF THE BATTLE

Simply knowing why you were born to run isn't enough to take you on the streets (or conveyor belt, as in the case of treadmills) and start running. Chances are, you'll need to be motivated to use that God-given trait. In the next chapter, I'll show you some of the best reasons why you should run. And believe me, they're worth it.

Chapter 2
Benefits of Running

People who take up running do it to either lose weight or to stay healthy. Running is the best form of exercise especially for people who want to reduce a few pounds without hitting the gym. It doesn't just provide good exercise for your body; it also helps in increasing stamina. Here are a few more reasons why running is beneficial.

Burns Calories

The first and foremost reason to take up running is the fact that it helps you burn calories faster and in a healthy manner. If you are the outdoorsy types, this is by far the best exercise that will help you burn the fat.

Running Makes You Feel Good

The feeling of exhilaration and high that you get from running are well worth the time and effort you make to run. It also boosts the serotonin levels in your brain, helping you relax and calm your mind. It's a great stress buster and good for your overall mental wellness.

Strong Lungs

One of the best and prolonged effects of running is strong lungs. As compared to most of types of exercising, running improves your lung capacity.

Curbs High Blood Pressure

Stop the blood pressure pills and wear your running shoes. Regular running expands and contracts your arteries, which helps in regulating your blood pressure (BP).

Improves Density of Your Bones

When you run for a long time, it puts stress on your bones. When your bones are put under stress, your body sends out essential minerals, which in turn makes them strong and improves their density. Not to forget the fact that you also get strong legs when you run regularly.

Easy and Cost Efficient Process

You don't need to pay anyone. You don't need any special gadgets, machines, or training. All you have to do is put your right foot forward then your left foot forward and repeat this process however long you want.

No Rigidity of Place

You can run in the park, in a field, on a track, on a hill, anywhere you want to run, you are free to do it. Then there is the good old treadmill if you are not particularly fond of the outdoors. As long as you have the will to run, you have a way to do it.

Effects Don't Stop Even After You Have

Various studies have found that the calorie burning effects of exercises like running, which have a high intensity, stay for a longer time when you've stopped the exercise as compared to the exercises that are of a lower intensity (for example: walking).

You Make a Better Use of Your Time

You burn more calories while running than you would if you were walking or doing an exercise of a lower intensity in the same amount of time.

James Sinclair

Chapter 3
How to Lose Weight By Running

Why We Get Fat

To enable you to understand how to lose weight effectively it is important to understand why we get fat in the first place. The whole world seems to be getting fat these days with doctors and scientists trying hard to find a solution. In reality the solution is quite simple.

Over the last few decades our diets have turned more and more towards processed foods. Our grandparents were a generation who would buy ingredients to make their food with. They would spend time in the kitchen preparing meals from scratch and they were generally healthy.

Did you know that during WWII in the UK people were healthier than they are today even though they were on rations?

The reason is because people were eating real food and very little else. You may have got hold of some sweets or chocolate but there was very little about. People would grow their own vegetables and could eat as much of that as they liked. With that diet people were lean and physically active.

Fast forward to the 21st century and we are for the most part living on processed food and are generally inactive.

So what is it about processed food that is so bad?

In short, processed food typically has several key differences from real food. Let us go through each difference one at a time.

Sugar

Sugar has been added to almost all processed food which is probably the biggest reason why people are getting fat. When you consume sugar your body increases insulin which in turn forces the energy from the food you have eaten into your fat cells. Basically you get fat.

Fiber

Another difference is that fiber in processed food is normally removed. It is the fiber that slows down the effects of sugar reducing the amount of insulin and ultimately reducing the amount of energy pushed into your fat cells.

In the real food that our grandparents would eat any food that had sugar, which was only fruits and vegetables, also had fiber. That meant there was never a problem.

Today sugar has been added to everything including many foods that you wouldn't expect there to be sugar in. Without the fiber our insulin levels remain high and our fat stores continue to grow.

In order to lose weight by running you need to get your eating right first. This means eating real food and cutting out the processed food that you are more than likely currently eating.

You can eat unprocessed meats, fish, eggs, nuts, fruits, and vegetables. If man has not played with it or created it then you can eat it.

What that will do is keep your insulin levels low to non existent. At that point your fat cells will be able to release the stored energy that can then be burnt as you run. The result will be weight loss through a reduced amount of fat - perfect.

You will however need to be aware of a few things that you could fall fowl of. It is what I call The Big Obesity Conspiracy.

The Big Obesity Conspiracy

For those who have not come across this term before let me tell you a little more about the Big Obesity Conspiracy. I go into more detail in my book but I will summarize it here. You need to know this to ensure you do not fall into the trap.

Food Industry

If you are overweight, then you are that way because of what you eat. All weight loss results from the food you eat. While many doctors will say you need to exercise more you can only do that if you eat the right foods.

Eating foods high in sugar as I have already explained will cause your insulin to rise and the energy you have eaten to go into your fat cells. You not only get fatter but you also have no energy left to use.

That means you don't feel like going for a run; you simply don't have the energy. Really you do have the energy but it is all trapped in your fat cells and cannot leave because your insulin levels are preventing it.

As long as you are on a highly processed diet you will not be able to lose weight and maintain it.

Diets

As a result of everyone eating a processed food diet and putting on weight, all sorts of diets have sprung up. There are hundreds of them all trying to reinvent the wheel.

There is everything from cutting out whole food groups, eating nothing but cabbage, drinking all your food, and even eating next to nothing for two days a week.

There are even slimming clubs that get you to buy their branded food disguised as healthy eating but in reality all you are doing is buying a different type of processed food.

Diets do not work; they never have and they never will. Do yourself a favor and stay well clear of them.

Exercise Equipment

Another way that companies will get money out of you on false promises is to get you to buy exercise equipment. This has become a million-dollar industry selling all sorts of items to tens of thousands of people each year, yet the population continues to get heavier by the year.

You may have purchased an exercise bike to use at home yourself. It has more than likely become a convenient place to hand your ironed shirts.

The problem with this method is it is still buying in to the 'burn more calories than you consume' paradigm. While you do need to burn more calories than you consume this only works if you keep your insulin low. It assumes that calories from sugar are the same as calories from everything else.

This industry sells products because people think they can just burn off the calories. As a wise man once said 'you cannot exercise off a bad diet'. You can however exercise off the fat when you are eating a good one.

Weight Loss Pills

Many people also invest in weight loss pills. This is again a bad move. As you now know, if you eat an unprocessed diet and exercise you will lose weight. Who needs pills?

Pills actually in many cases have side effects, none of which involve losing weight and keeping it off in the long run. They will however result in you losing a whole load of your hard earned cash.

In conclusion, the way to eat is to eat fresh unprocessed foods that are low in sugar and high in fiber. I am talking about meat, fish, eggs, nuts, fruits, and vegetables. Eat them and exercise and you WILL lose weight.

Calorie Mathematics

Ok so now that you know that eating right and exercise will result in weight loss, we need to do the mathematics behind it.

Each pound of fat no matter where it is on your body has a total of 3500 calories. This means that if you need to lose 10 pounds in weight you simply multiply 3500 by 10, giving 35,000. So to lose that much weight you need to burn 35,000 more calories than you consume. Simple enough isn't it?

Once you have the number of calories you need to lose you can work out how many you want to lose a day. To keep things simple let us say it is 500 a day; that would mean you would lose 1 pound a week. You can then set your food and exercise accordingly.

It is calories burnt minus calories consumed to give you your weight loss. Calories burnt are a total of active metabolic rate and exercise combined.

You start this by working out your active metabolic rate. Now you may have heard of basic metabolic rate but you may not have heard of active. Let me explain.

In case you don't know, Basic Metabolic Rate will give you the number of calories your body will burn each day just keeping you alive. It assumes you do nothing but exist.

Active metabolic rate takes into account the fact that you get out of bed, you may go up and down stairs, do the hovering, go to work and so on.

Knowing how many calories you burn in a day can never be 100% but you can get it close.

When I was losing weight I used the calculations found in one of Jillian Michaels books. It can also be found on her website. It allows you to work out what you burn each day. See below.

Basic Metabolic Rate (BMR)

Males = 66 + (6.23 x body weight in pounds) + (12.7 x height in inches) − (6.8 x age in years)

Female = 655 + (4.3 x weight in pounds) + (4.7 x height in inches) − (4.7 x age in years)

This will give you your basic metabolic rate or the number of calories you need just to stay alive.

Active Metabolic Rate (AMR)

To work out your active metabolic rate you now need to take the basic metabolic rate and multiply it by one of the numbers below depending on which one applies to you.

1.1 – Sedentary Physical Activity

1.2 – Light Physical Activity

1.3 – Moderate Physical Activity

1.4 – High Physical Activity

Once you have your Active Metabolic Rate (AMR) number you can begin to work out how many calories you can burn in a day. You now need to add the number of calories burnt through running to the AMR and that's your daily burn. Simply subtract the amount of calories eaten through food and you have your calorie burn for the day.

We have often heard that running is the best form of exercising. The truth is not far from it. Running is definitely one of the best ways to lose weight and one of the healthiest options for the wellbeing of your body. However, it is not as simple as it seems. You need to focus your energy in the right manner towards running if you want to get the best results.

How to Increase Fat Loss With Running

Instead of a slow, steady, and long run all the time, run at a slow pace for about a minute and then increase the intensity for about half a minute. Repeat this many times during your run. This way, fat loss will be increased.

If you are running on a flat road or ground, try running on some inclined area or hill. You will burn more calories and lose more fat. Run up the incline for a few seconds, rest a few seconds and jog back. If you have no hill in your vicinity, then you can use the treadmill for this purpose at a 5% incline for a few seconds. Then set it back to normal for some time. Repeat it a few times.

Run up stairs and return back jogging slowly. This helps in fat loss.

Mostly runners run about twice a week or a maximum of 4 times a week. This is not sufficient for fat loss or weight loss. If you run more often, your metabolic activity is increased and you burn more calories, resulting in more fat loss. You will also be a better runner this way. Fat loss should be gradual. This helps you perform better.

If you are a new runner, then start with short runs. Gradually increase the distance and intensity. Start off your eating for weight loss simultaneously by first stopping all the extra calories you are consuming. Start having nutritious food to improve your health. Reduce the quantity of the food you have been eating until now. Replace all the junk food or high calorie food with nutritious and lower calorie foods.

For experienced runners, it is not possible to lose weight by increasing their intensity slowly as they are already into intense training. They can increase their running by 4-5 miles per session. It might help them to lose weight.

Improving Body Composition

You may have heard this many times, but let me educate you again, weight loss is not all about exercise; you need to watch what you eat too. So if you want to get the maximum benefits from running, you need to focus on your diet too. Maintain a food dairy wherein you record the details of what you eat, how much you eat, and the calorie content of that food. Plan your meals a day earlier, just as you plan your running (time, distance, etc.). Eat right and take good care of yourself.

Body composition of regular runners can be improved through diet. Runners have to reduce the amount of fat in their diet in order to lose weight and improve their body composition. Fat helps gain weight in runners so cut down on fats. This in turn makes you lean. Every gram of fat has more than twice the amount of calories that is present in a gram of carbohydrate or protein.

Fat is absorbed faster as compared to proteins or carbohydrates. Less energy is spent to process fat. Weight loss takes place only when the daily intake reduces. So in other words, if you as a runner reduce or remove rich fat food from your daily diet, the calories are automatically reduced and you have high chances of losing weight. You can replace the rich fats with low fat products that have lesser calories.

Remember not to eliminate it totally. Only reduce it. If you eliminate it totally, you will end up with vitamin and mineral deficiencies. Try to have monounsaturated fats and omega-3 fats as much as possible. So if you plan your diet carefully, weight loss can take place.

At times people want rapid weight loss and end up eating about 900-1000 calories on a daily basis. Since you will be reducing your total calorie intake, naturally your carbohydrate intake will also be low. Because of this the glycogen stored in the muscle gets depleted. Due to the glycogen depletion from the muscles, runners are not able to give quality outputs. There are signs of fatigue and feeling less competitive. This leads to health problems like losing body protein, electrolytes getting imbalanced, you becoming dehydrated, etc. This is not a sensible way, so follow a good diet.

Chapter 4
How to Reduce The Risk of Injury

The Dilemma of Foot Injury

It is common to find that a lot of people suffer from foot injuries. While there can be various reasons for being inured, one of the common ones among them has to be the problem with foot strike.

Those who are not aware of the ideal ways by which they should place their foot should get familiar with the best foot strike method. Not only will it help you in avoiding injuries, but at the same time, it is also going to offer you the right head start regarding how to maximize the output from running activities.

Maximize Your Potential

When you are aware of the best foot strike methods, you will be able to maximize your running potential. When you are running, it is important to get to your potential. While there are exercises that help in improving the potential, a lot of it depends upon the running posture as well. So, you need to learn the right foot strike method such that you will be able to cover longer distances much more effectively.

Now that you are aware of the reasons, you need to learn the best foot strike. So, let us get ahead and learn the finest foot strike ways that you can follow.

Foot strike refers to the mechanism of how and where the foot makes contact with the ground when you are running. When you are running, whether it is consciously, or subconsciously, different parts of your foot can come in contact with the ground,impacting the way you run and the benefits you get from it.

There are three main styles of foot strike, namely:

- Heel

- Mid foot

- Toe

Runners can use either of these three foot strikes and we will explain each one of them here.

The Heel Foot Strike

This is the posture when you are running and it is your heel that touches the ground. Following are the benefits that you will reap from it.

This is perhaps the most natural form of running and so the strain that you will experience is going to be very minimal. Those who want to run really long distances can benefit immensely from this form of foot strike. It also helps in stretching the calf muscles so you will be able to ensure smoother running and it can help in thinning of thigh muscles as well.

However, there are a few issues with this foot strike method too. It is extremely easy to over stride and the knees and hips will find extra load that can sometimes lead to injuries as well. Further, sometimes you will find that your running may be a little slow because your heels will act like brakes every time you take a stride and they make contact with the ground.

The Mid Foot Strike

It is good for those who want to pace up their running speed. The time duration for which the foot is on the ground is lessened and thus you will be able to sprint a lot faster. Not only this, if you are worried about the shock absorption in your joints, you will find this foot strike method to be apt.

However, when you are learning the mid foot strike method, you will find a little bit of unease. It is mostly not a natural way to run and people need time to get adjusted to running this way. You also need to be careful with the Achilles heel and the calf muscles because they will be under a lot of strain.

The Toe Strike

When you choose to have a toe strike, you will be able to sprint a lot faster. The emphasis on your knees and ankles are going to be significantly less. However, the amount of energy that your body spends when it uses the toe strike is much higher and so you may get tired very soon.

It is important to note that there is no one method that can be termed as the best foot strike. You need to improvise the foot strike method based upon what you are looking for. Different people may be comfortable with varying movements and so based upon your health, ease, comfort, and other factors, you can choose whichever foot strike seems to be best for you.

When you are more concerned about your speed, it is the toe strike that seems to be most apt for you. However, if you want to run naturally and sprint with ease, the heel foot strike seems to be the best choice you have.

So, try out each of the different ways and pick the ideal foot strike methods to maximize your running output.

Every runner is at a risk of getting injured. The aim of every runner should be to avoid getting injured. Don't rush. Do everything slowly. If you are a beginner, do not run too much. If you run too much you are bound to get injured. For a start, you should not run for more than 9

– 10 miles per week. Give time for muscle repair and joint repair.

Experts have devised a plan on how you should go about with your running. In the first week, run no more than 10 miles. In the second week, make it 11 miles. In the third week, make it 12 miles, and so on and so forth. In simple words, increase your running speed gradually. Just in case you have get injured in spite of gradually increasing your run, then give time for injury repair. Do not be in a hurry to get back to your old routine. Give time to heal. Don't hurry.

Your body sends you signals if you are over-doing something. The signs are aches, constant pain, etc. Do not ignore these signals. If you continue you are bound to get injured. Consult your doctor. Find out the cause of the pain. Seek out the proper medication or physiotherapy.

When you feel the first sign, do not run for 3-4 days. Take a rest day. Then start off with walking on the second day. Increase your walk on the third day or do some swimming or cycling. If your pain does not persist, then you can start running on the fourth day. You must run as well as walk. Increase gradually. Do not overdo it. If the pain persists, then visit your doctor.

If you have joint pain or muscle pain, then the best thing that works is rest and ice packs for immediate treatment. Ice packs reduce inflammation of the muscles. You can make your own ice pack at home by putting a few cubes of ice along with chilled water in a plastic bag. Doctors suggest elevation as immediate treatment. For example, if your leg is injured, place your leg in an elevated position. Next you can compress the problem area with a bandage. Wait until you are heeled. Don't hurry.

Strength training should be used to balance your body. Keep your body aligned. Strengthen your hip muscles. If you have a knee injury, then strengthen the hip muscles. When you strengthen the hip muscles, the stability of your legs is increased right up to your ankle. If your muscle balance is not proper, then you start having problems.

Do not run on uneven surfaces. Always run on a leveled surface. In case you have no leveled surface, it is better to run on the treadmill. Treadmill running is good for those who are recovering from injury. It is less risky than running on uneven surfaces.

Do not run at too high of a speed. This is one of the greatest risks in getting injured. If you are back from an injury, be all the more careful. You are at a higher risk.

Stretch the muscles at the back of your legs, the hamstring and calf muscles. This way the knee movement is improved. If the calf muscles are flexible, then the Achilles tendon and plantar fascia will remain healthy.

Wear proper shoes. Wrong shoes can cause injury. See that the soles are not worn out. If so, it is time you get a new pair of shoes.

Fixes for Bad Running Form

Zipper Lines

Running is a kind of sport. A lot of runners use up a lot of energy winding their upper bodies, fighting the lower body's efforts. Imagine the zipper line of a jacket running down the midpoint of your upper body. When your hands cross the zipper line, the top half of the body and the shoulders would normally follow your hands. The twisting made from the midriff up is energy that can be used for you to run faster.

Notice your hands' position as they swing while you are running. When you look at your forefinger and thumb, you will notice that your hands are likely crossing the line of the zipper. A small adjustment is all that you need. Hold your hands a bit broader from the body, a bit broader than your hips. As the arm swings back, try to reach into the back of your pocket. It spreads your reach further in a straighter line with less crossing of the zipper line.

Chicken Wings

When we are tired, our arm posture changes and the position of the body, especially the arms, would normally become similar to the wings of chickens. The shoulders would go up closer to the ears, as if we're shrugging and keeping that shrug as we run. Similar to a chicken, we cannot fly properly with our arms held firmly to both sides of our body. This results to shorter arm swing and shorter step as we run. When we do more strides, we are using more energy that covers the distance to our goal.

Pain in the shoulders and the neck are the first signs of running with chicken wings. If you keep getting this kind of discomfort, then you should check if you are still in the right form. Try to relax your shoulders and drop your arms on your side and run by shaking your hands a bit. By doing this, you will release the stress you feel in your shoulders and neck.

Potato Chips

This common inefficiency happens when we tighten our hands into firmly held fists. The tension in our forearms goes up to the shoulders and spreads to the other parts of the body. This tension makes our hearts beat harder to thrust oxygen-rich blood into the muscles, and it results in more misused energy and, eventually, makes us run slower.

In order to release this kind of tension, imagine holding a potato chip and not breaking it. If your hands are compressed so firmly that you cannot hold that chip, jiggle your fingers and release your grip. The tension of the body will reverse and it will allow the release of more oxygen-rich blood to the muscles with every beat of the heart. We will go back to a longer, smoother, more effective stride, and more energy will be saved for the final kick.

Always pay attention to your running form as this will help you to reach your goal easier.

James Sinclair

Chapter 5

The Essential Dynamics of Running

When you are running with the main motive of losing weight, you need to have the right kind of regime to follow. Running is all about choosing the right style, posture, and form.

There are too many points you will have to bear in mind and some of the main ones among them are as follows.

• Remember, speed is not everything when you run. Obviously, if you are merely sauntering at a leisurely pace, you are less likely to lose weight. However, what you need to know is that there are other things that trigger weight loss too. So, you will have to learn about those points, focus on them, and then work your way towards better running for greater weight loss.

• The duration of your running time is important. However, you should not end up exhausting your body. You have to be aware of the amount of exhaustion your body can handle. Further, interval training is often considered to be a much more effective method for the sake of losing weight. Rather than concentrating mainly upon running for long hours, you can break your running duration into shorter, but multiple bursts. Those who are not familiar with the interval training method need to know that it is a form of training wherein you carry out profuse exercises at your uppermost limit for a short duration of time. After this, you will either let your body relax completely or else you can lessen the intensity considerably which allows your body to relax and the muscles can gain back their strength. Once you have done so, you can once again resume your high intensity exercises all over again. This way you can alternate high and low intensity exercises and trigger greater weight loss.

• Do you have a complete workout? Even though you may be merely running, it is important to ensure that you have a systematic workout wherein you know when to run, the forms of running to choose, the duration of your jog, and the days you can take a rest as well. There are different kinds of running routines available and you should choose the ones that are best suited for your body and schedule.

The Best Running Program

When you are looking to make the most out of your urge to run and shed the extra pounds, you will need the right kind of running program. This is why you will have to follow a systematic and disciplined approach.

Walking and Running Go Hand in Hand

You need to incorporate walking into your running program. When you want to shed the extra pounds and get the perfect body figure, you should ideally start with a 2 minute walk. When you are walking, all your muscles will get loosened up and they will be all set to take up the strain of running. Now, when you start your running regime, you need to understand the foot strike that you must use. You should pick the right kind of foot strike that is apt for your own style.

Ideally, it is best advised to carry a timer to keep track of how long you should run. When you are running, the time of your running regime is important. You have to push your body in order to lose weight with running. Let your metabolism accelerate and your muscles must be tired. It is when the extra calories are burned that you will be able to shed the extra pounds. Burning of fat isn't the easiest of processes and so you will have to keep working hard, and despite the fact that it won't be easy, keep on following this regime.

You need to push your body a little more every day. Every day, before you begin your running, you need to be aware of what you have already achieved. Before starting the running exercises, have your eyes set on improving your target goals. You must aspire to run more than what you have already managed to cover yesterday. It is this attitude that is going to help you in losing a lot more weight.

When you are running, you need to be sure that you are comfortable with your running style. Do not try too hard as this will prevent you from running naturally and it is only going to add to your hassles rather than being of help. Whichever running style you pick, make sure to follow it consistently such that you will have the right set of rewards to reap.

Distance Isn't Everything

While it is important to be mindful of the amount of distance you are covering, merely emphasizing on distance is not going to be sufficient. When you want to lose weight with the help of running, you have to look at other factors too.

Look at your stride length, the duration for which you are training, and the time when you train. Mostly, running early in the morning on an empty stomach is going to offer you the best set of rewards. The rate of burning of calories is going to be highest when you are running early in the morning. Sometimes you may lack the motivation which is needed to run and in these cases, you will have to work hard and try and motivate yourself because staying fit has a lot of perks to offer.

When you are running, your body muscles will flex and the stress that is put on your body means that the metabolic rate is going to speed up as well. This helps in burning a lot more calories so you will be able to shed the extra pounds as well. The faster you run, the more calories you are likely to burn.

Running Outside Vs. Treadmill

It's almost impossible to find a gym that doesn't have a treadmill, and a lot of people go to the gym to run on the treadmill. But why do many people just run outside instead of paying for the gym just to run on the treadmill?

Most of the time, you'll hear stories about how running outdoors is a heavy activity for many people that can lead to damage of the knees. While treadmills on the other hand, are cushioned to absorb the impact of every step, making it safer. You can also run on it regardless of the weather. With the treadmill you are running on an even surface and you do not need to think about your safety from drivers or bumping other people on the street.

Does this make you think that the treadmill is better than running outside? Let's take a deeper look...

What is Happening When We Run?

First of all, we spread a leg out in front with our thigh muscles before bringing the foot down and making contact with the ground. At this time, your muscles conquest pulling and bending the leg to push us through as the other leg spreads out to do the sequence again.

So to put it simply, we're always doing leg extensions followed by curling of legs, moving the muscles on two sides of your legs.

But this is not the case on the treadmill. Yes, we are still extending our legs but it is limited to the treadmill belt taking over instead of pushing our bodies onward with the following leg muscles, the belt performs this by dragging the foot towards the back. Basically, when it comes to the leg muscles, we're doing half of the work and are just using the frontal muscles to do it.

It means that less calories are burned because of fewer muscles being used and furthermore, the imbalance can lead to stress, mainly on the knee.

It goes slightly in contradiction of the argument that running on a treadmill is safer than running outdoors when it comes to joint matters.

Additionally, research performed by the University of East London in 1998 claims that the hip flexion angle rises considerably when we run on a treadmill. Knee and hip flexion angles need to upturn in order to carry the hip through the pace leading to a jerking and exhaustion of your hip flexor muscles. Because of this, method changes automatically in order to pawn this weakness leading you to have bad form. It could also lead to knee pain, compounding the problem of the unnecessary muscle growth.

Experts have also seen that once your foot steps on the treadmill belt, the ankle, foot, and shin become momentarily a part of the treadmill belt and move rearward from the central body mass at similar speed. It means that the bone in the shin isn't as straight as it would be on a normal run and is forced into a larger range of movement that sequentially can cause stress to both the bone and the muscles it supports, leading to a tight feeling called shin splints.

It doesn't mean that you completely have to avoid running on the treadmill. Running on the treadmill for occasional cardiovascular workout is very beneficial.

Furthermore, throughout the winter or rainy season, running outdoors is not pleasant, so going for a treadmill run would be the best alternative if you don't want to lose your progression.

To put it briefly, treadmills surely have their place, but if you have the chance, it's always better to run outside and enjoy the sight at the same time. There is a big world out there you can discover while running, places and thing that you might be missing in your daily commutes. Give your lungs some fresh air while enjoying the Vitamin D from the sun, and all other benefits you can get from running on the road.

James Sinclair

Chapter 6
Warming Up and Cooling Off

The first basic rule of exercise, which applies to running as well - Always do a warm-up before running and cool off after finishing your run.

Guide to Warming Up

One should always do a little warm activity before running. Why? A nice warm up expands your blood vessels, which in turn increases the intake of oxygen. The increased intake of oxygen helps raise the temperature of your muscles and makes them more flexible and efficient. Since the warm up increases your heart rate slowly, the stress of the exercise on your heart also decreases.

Steps to Warm Up

To ensure that you have warmed up correctly, try these easy exercises. They are perfect whether you are running for 5km or 50km. The great thing about these warm up routines is that you only need around 20 meters of space in front of you to execute them properly.

High Skips

This exercise is similar to skipping but without a rope, although you are aiming to gain more height. As you jump upwards, concentrate on raising your knee in an upward motion on each jump. Start with your left leg and alternate as you proceed. You might need to use the opposite arm to help stabilize yourself, especially if you jump fairly high.

Butt Kicks

Slowly move forward in a straight line and starting with your left foot flick backwards so that your heel connects with your butt. Start off slowly, alternating between your left and right feet, building up speed as you go along until you are performing the warm up fairly quickly. Try to focus on making sure your heel strikes your butt on every kick.

High Knees

This exercise is a 180-degree reversal of the butt kick. Here you want to bring your needs up towards your chest, starting with your left foot and alternating as you move slowly forward. Again, you want to focus on achieving a fairly decent speed executing the exercise. Do not worry about how much distance you move forward. Repeat this 10 times for each leg.

Walking Lunges

These are similar to a lunge except you will be walking forward slowly. Take a step with your left leg. Slowly begin to lower your frame downwards. The object is to make a 90-degree angle between your left leg (the front) and your right leg (the back). When you do this correctly, the knee of your front leg will be straight over your ankle. Move slowly upwards and repeat but this time with your right leg. Do this 10 times in total.

Frankenstein

Place your arms out in front of you at 90 degrees to your body. Starting with your left leg, kick in an upward motion. You need to aim to hit your palm of your left hand with your left toe, keeping your leg as straight as possible, and your toes pointed upwards. Alternate to your right leg. Do 15 kicks for each leg.

Leg Swings

You will need something to support you when doing these exercises. Start by holding onto a wall with your right hand while beginning to swing your opposite leg. First swing forward, return to your starting position and then swing it backwards. Concentrate on making each swing a full motion without any pauses. Try and swing the leg as far forward or as far backwards as it can possibly go. Do 15 swings for each leg before changing to swinging each leg in a similar motion, but this time across the body.

What About Stretching?

Although these warm up routines should be more than adequate to set you up for your run, some runners also like to incorporate a stretching routine before they run. Here are a few stretches that you can try. Repeat each of these three times. You will need a wall to perform some of them.

Calf Stretch

Face the wall and place your arms out in front of you. Place your palms upwards against the wall while keeping your feet flat on the ground around a shoulder length apart. Now slowly lean forward with your hips. As you do this, start to bend your knees a little. You will begin to feel your calves stretch as you do this.

Lower Calf Stretch

Bend your body forward, keeping your palms in an upright position against the wall (your body should be roughly 90 degrees to the wall). Move your left foot forward and bend your knee slightly. Slowly lift your left foot upwards. You will begin to feel your lower calf stretch as you do this. Repeat with your right leg.

Triceps and Shoulder Stretch

Standing tall, take hold of your left elbow with your right hand. Begin to pull your elbow towards your body. You will feel your triceps and shoulder begin to stretch as you do this. Repeat with your right elbow.

Hamstring Stretch

Stand upright, bend forward and touch your toes, moving up and down slowly by no more than 10 centimeters. You will begin to feel your hamstrings stretch as you do this.

Quadriceps Stretch

Face the wall, stand on your right foot only using the wall to balance. Now hold your right foot with your left hand behind you. Begin to pull the foot towards your buttocks. You will begin to feel your quadriceps stretch as you do this. Repeat with your right leg.

Groin Stretch

Sit on the ground and place your feet together but with the soles of your shoes touching each other. Now place your elbows on your knees and slowly begin to lean forward. Use your elbows to press your knees towards the ground. You will begin to feel your groin stretch as you do this.

Now you are ready to tackle anything the road or trail can throw at you!

Guide to Cooling Off

Cooling off after running is also an essential activity. Suddenly halting after a good run makes your blood pressure and heart rate fall suddenly and can make you feel light headed. Cooling off helps them drop slowly.

Steps to Cooling Off

Cooling down routine helps the muscles, and the body for that matter, return to a normal state. Your heart rate, as well as your breathing, will slow down as your core body temperature drops. A proper cool down also performs the following very important functions.

Stops Blood From Pooling

While running, the muscles in our legs contract, sending blood back to our heart for it to once again pump it back through our bodies. If you just stop after completing a run, blood can begin to pool in your legs as your muscles have stopped contracting. This leads to a massive drop in blood pressure, dizziness, or sometimes fainting in very extreme cases. By cooling down, your body resumes normal operation naturally.

Helps to Remove Lactic Acid Build Up

While we exercise, lactic acid builds up in our muscles. By using a warming down routine, lactic acid is removed from the muscles.

Reduces Levels of Adrenaline

While running, the body releases adrenaline raising our heart rate, blood pressure, and breathing rate. Warming down helps to remove this adrenaline from our system, thus helping with the body's recovery rate.

Aids Muscle Recovery

Lastly, by warming down properly, you allow your muscles to recover faster, reducing the risk of injury in future running sessions.

Form and Technique: How to Run

The key to maximizing your speed as well as your distance when you run is your form. Running with the proper form can also protect you from injuries and give you a better physical and mental workout. If you run the wrong way, you're going to get into bad habits that are hard to break. Pay attention to your form, and use a few techniques while you're running to ensure that you're doing it properly.

Your running technique will depend on your size, strength, and flexibility. What works for one runner won't necessarily work for every runner and you need to make sure you're focused on comfort and safety. If you remember these important techniques, you'll be sure to run correctly.

Pushing up and off the ground is the way you want to start and maintain a stride. Think of leaving the ground behind you as you run in order to ensure that your feet are doing what they need to do to keep the rest of your body moving.

Keep your stride short and fast. You don't want to do any leaping. You also don't want to think about distance right now. Take short, fast steps while you run in order to find the right pace and keep good form.

Put your foot right below your knee. The leg should be in a straight line, with the foot coming down onto the ground right underneath where your knee is located. If your foot is reaching out in front of where your knee is, you're setting yourself up for a potential injury. Don't worry about toe/heel or heel/toe. It doesn't matter which part of your foot hits the ground first, as long as it's lined up under your knee.

Bend your elbows. If you've ever seen anyone running with their arms straight down by their sides, you know it looks weird. It's also counterproductive to running for exercise. Bend your elbows and hold them at your sides at 90 degree angles.

Keep your head and your chest up, ensuring that you aren't bending over at the waist. Hold your shoulders back and keep your eyes focused on what's ahead of you. Let your hands relax. You don't want to ball them into fists or let them flail around while you run. They should be loose and level with your midsection.

Running for Beginners - The Walking – Running - Walking Method

If you are a newbie at running or exercising, you are going to have difficulty in running for long stretches of time at the initial stages of your running regime. We recommend the walking-running-walking method for you. It is very simple and reduces the chances of injury.

Once you're done with your warm up, start by taking a walk. After a few minutes of walking, run for a short while then slow down into a walk again after a few minutes. Start with walking more and running less at first then you can gradually increase the time intervals and walking-running spans. Keep repeating this until you can run for long stretches of time. Remember to always begin with walking and then transition into running. It helps your muscles to adjust properly. If you start running suddenly, it will make you feel drained out once you slow down. Your walk should not be a slow walk either, take long strides with your posture correct. Your walking speed should be fast enough to keep your heart rate levels from falling too much. It is not advisable to cool down fully then run again and then cool down fully again.

It is important to set certain goals like the distance you want to cover in a particular amount of time and try to follow through with it as much as you can. If you feel a little tired by the end, slow down but do not stop until you have reached your goal. It is your determination and will power that is going to help you lose those extra inches of flab on your tummy and hips.

Chapter 7

Running- The Framework and Postures

Like any other activity, even running has a proper form. Perfecting your running postures can help increase your speed, efficiency, and minimize the risk of injury and stress on your body. Here are a few helpful tips to follow while running:

Tips for Your Feet

Do not run on your toes or heels. If you run on your toes, you might feel exhausted very quickly and may develop a pain in your shin. If run on your heels, it may cause you injury and causes a loss in energy. When your feet strike the ground, let the middle of your foot be the part that touches the ground first and then the toes.

You should also keep your toes pointed straight in front, toward the direction you are running. Clenching your toes in can sometimes make you fall or injure yourself. Try not to stop suddenly in the middle of a run.

Tips for Your Hands

Let your hands and arms be at ease while running. Holding your hands near your chest will make you feel tired more quickly. Let them relax and keep them at the side, somewhere near your waist and hips. Try not to clench your fists while running. It can cause a slight rigidness in the neck and arm muscles. Do not swing your arms from the elbow; instead swing them from the shoulder joint.

Correct Your Posture

Keep your head, shoulders, and back as straight as possible while running. Do not jerk your shoulders while running and do not let them reach or go above your ears. Keep checking your posture at regular intervals. Do not slump. Slumping can lead to back and shoulder pains. Keep your shoulders relaxed and level. Do not slouch or hunch your shoulders over, it can hamper your breathing.

Breathing Techniques

While you are running, you should breathe through your mouth as well as nose. When you breathe through your mouth, you get more oxygen. Just nose breathing is insufficient to get the oxygen you need.

Do belly breathing instead of chest breathing. With belly breathing, you are inhaling more oxygen. While breathing in, inhale through your nose. Breathe in fully. While breathing out, exhale through your mouth. This way you are exhaling more carbon dioxide. Exhale fully.

Every time you inhale, try to take 3 foot strikes and as you exhale, try to take 2 foot strikes. Run at such a pace that you are at ease while running. Do not gasp. If you feel short of breath, then slow down or walk for a while. You will slowly feel better while breathing. Resume your running only when you feel fine.

Mindful Running: Getting the Most from Your Exercise

Naturally, most people run for the physical benefits. There is a lot to be gained for your heart health, weight management, and overall health when you adopt a consistent running routine. However, there are also a number of mental and emotional benefits to running. Not only can you beat back the potential for depression and stress, you can also use your running time to get in touch with your inner self and to increase your mindfulness. Being mindful while you run can help you sort out problems, using your subconscious to be present in the moment and focused on the really important things you have going on inside your mind and body.

Mindful running can happen naturally if you pay attention to a few key things. First, focus on your breathing. Inhale through your nose if you can, and allow your breathing to fall into the same pattern as your steps. The result will be meditative. Once your breathing is synced, look at your stride. Pay attention to how your feet look, sound, and feel. Visualize yourself being pulled forward as you run, and let your mind get quiet while you find your balance and your inner peace. This is mindful running and you'll find even better stress reduction benefits when you exercise this way.

Finding Motivation

The most important thing you need to run is the will or the motivation to actually get out there and do it. Some people may find the will to improve the way they look and find back their lost confidence from within. On the other hand, there are a few others who need to be pushed into getting out of the house and running.

If you are not motivated enough, you will find reasons to bail on running, so the best bet is to find a 'buddy runner' who has similar goals like you. You can both seek motivation from each other when you don't feel like running.

It is also important to set specific goals on how much you want to run in a week or month. Also set a goal about the number of pounds you want to lose in a specific time period. Your goals should be realistic ones that you actually have the ability to complete. Setting unrealistic goals can lower your confidence if you are not able to complete them, hence making you lose interest in running.

James Sinclair

Chapter 8
Preparing For Your First Race

Running in a race is a good way for you to access the social benefits of running. While a race usually indicates that you're competing against a field of other runners, you're not really competing against them as much as you're competing with them. Your goal should not really be to win the race (although that would be wonderful). Your goal is to improve your own personal best. Steadily improving your recorded running time is a great reason to enter races. Many people enjoy running in races to feel like part of a team or even to raise money for charity. Whatever your reasons for running in a race, you need to prepare yourself. If you're wondering how to train for your first race, the answer is fairly simple: you practice.

Choosing a Race

First, you need to choose the right race. Take a look at the distance first. The most common type of road race is the 5K, and it works well for beginners as well as experienced runners. If you have been running for a long time and you're finally ready to start entering races, you might be okay in a 10K. That's your own decision, but make sure you're choosing a distance that you're likely to finish. The only way not to win a race is by not crossing the finish line.

In addition to looking at distance, you need to consider the race route. If there are a lot of hills and uneven terrain, you need to be prepared for it. You also need to be prepared for weather; running a 5K in Miami in August will be a lot different than running in New York in January. Your first race should be in a place that feels familiar to you. One of the best things about running races is that you get to go to new places. However, for your first race you want to feel comfortable with the climate, terrain, and the general area that you'll be covering.

How to Train for Your First Race

Assuming you decide to run a 5K for starters, you'll need to work your way up to running at least that distance in one single outing. If your running progression has only led you to completing a mile or two, you're going to have to increase what you run on a daily basis. The 5K race you enter will equal just over three miles. If you're not sure you can run three miles every day - that's okay. It doesn't mean you can't run in a 5K race. You don't have to run that distance every day, you simply have to run it one day - on the race day. However, you want to enter the race with the confidence that you can complete it.

As you're training, run at least three miles one day per week. Even if you only run one mile three days a week, try to get that three mile run in on one day of the week. If you practice getting through the full three miles once a week, you'll know you can do it. Leading up to the race, follow your same training schedule. And if you do most of your running on a treadmill, get outside during the three mile run day so you'll be better prepared on race day.

Whether you run a 5K or a 10K or something in between, you'll enjoy the sense of accomplishment and community. Training simply means practicing, and if you practice your running on a consistent basis, you'll be ready. Track your time and try to improve with every race you win.

Chapter 9

Tips for Running Safely

Every runner should take precautions while running. Even though running is easy, there may be instances where you might end up getting injured, sometimes even severely. Your safety is the most important; hence here are a few safety tips that every runner must follow:

Inform Someone of Your Whereabouts

Before you start your run, take a couple of minutes for yourself. Check your shoes to see if the laces are secure and not hanging lose. Do not forget to inform a family member or a friend that you are going out for a run. At least one person should know where you are and what route you are taking so that they know where to look in case of an emergency. Carry your cell phone with you if possible, and keep your emergency contacts on speed dial.

Look in Front of You

You should look in front of you while running. A lot of people tend to look at the ground while running. It is not the safest way. If you are running in a well populated area with a lot of rush, you never know what might suddenly come in front of you.

Run Against the Traffic

If you are running on or near a road, it is better for you to run against the traffic. (Though, for your own safety, it is better to run off the road, especially if there is fast moving traffic.) It makes it easy for you to see the vehicles coming towards you. The drivers of the vehicles are able to spot you easily too.

Wear Bright Clothes/Luminous Gadgets

If possible, wear brightly colored clothes like a white or a yellow top that makes it easy for others to spot you from a distance. If you are running at dawn or dusk or at night, wear some reflective gear so that you are visible to others. They can be shoes, jackets, head-bands, T-shirts, wrist bands, or anything that sticks out enough to make people spot you easily in the dark.

Carry Your Identification with You

Carry your identification with you when you are running, be it a drivers license or your medical insurance card. You can also wear or carry an identity card that mentions important contact numbers in case of any emergency. There are utility belts available in the market that can hold cell phone and identification cards and any other gadgets or wallets that you may need to carry with you.

Pay Attention While Running

Try not to carry an iPod with you. It is advisable to run without music as it can cause distractions. You may not be able to hear the vehicles on the roads. Pay attention to the vehicles on the road and keep a safe distance. You should also pay attention to the people around you and make sure there are no shady characters about. If you feel something is off, trust your instincts and change direction to a safer place.

Be in Safe Areas

It is better to run in parks or running paths or in places where there are a lot of people. Run in an area you know well and aren't in danger of getting lost.

Tips for Runners Over 50

There is nothing called a 'right age' when it comes to running, exercising, cycling, and swimming. Anyone can run. Running is one healthy exercise for all age groups.

1. Consult your doctor before you start off. Have a medical checkup and get the necessary tests done. Go ahead when your doctor gives you the green signal.

2. Do not run alone. Go with some company or a group of runners. Have your identification and medical insurance card with you at all times. Keep cash and ATM card with you.

3. You may not be able to run as well as you did in your 20's, 30's, and 40's. It is never too late. Slow down. Take rest in between your running. Set realistic goals. Your legs may hurt. Slow down, rest for a while, and start again. Start at a slow speed and gradually increase as the days pass by. When you do not feel like running

you can take up any other activity like swimming, cycling, light walking, etc.

James Sinclair

Chapter 10
Running Gear and Dressing

Running Shoes

Buy a good pair of running shoes from a good store that deals with running shoes. There are generally experts available to guide you in these types of shoe stores. They will guide you into buying the type of shoe that suits your style of running and size of foot. They are different from walking shoes. Try the shoes on. You should have at least a gap equal to 1 finger between your big toe and the end of the shoe.

Running Socks

You should buy at least 3-4 pairs of good quality running socks. Do not wear cotton socks as it absorbs the sweat leaving you uncomfortable. It can cause blisters in summer and you will feel cold in winters. So wear socks that are synthetic.

Utility Belt

You should own a utility belt so that all important and necessary things will fit in it like ATM card, identity card, cash, important phone numbers, water bottles, some energy drink in case of dehydration, a little bit of first aid, etc.

Running Watch

Ideally, you should own a running watch; it helps you time your runs. There are some running watches that have GPS tracking, while some of them can track your heart rate. Invest in a good one that caters to your needs.

Running Glares

Protect your eyes from the UV rays of the sun with a good pair of running glares that are able to block the UV rays. It will protect your eyes from dust, insects, and hot or cold wind.

Sports Bra

If you are a woman, you need a high impact sports bra. Opt for a decent brand of sports bra that will provide support to your bust areas, help your skin breathe, and not trap in the sweat.

Log Book

Maintain a log book. Keep a record of your runs, the routes you have taken, the number of rest days, etc.

Sippers or Water Bottles

In spite of the cold weather, you sweat while running. So keep yourself hydrated. Drink lots of water or sports drink. Keep yourself well hydrated.

Dressing

The type of clothes you wear while running is essential or it can end up being a very uncomfortable run for you. Do not wear tight fitting clothes. Wear loose fitting clothes that are light colored. This will help your body breathe. Do not wear cotton clothes as it will wick moisture away from the skin. You feel hotter in dark colored clothes as dark colors absorb sunlight and heat. Wear clothes that are made of synthetic fabric. Dress up properly whatever the weather is.

What to Wear in Hot Weather While Running

Wear loose fitting synthetic clothes because it wicks moisture away from your skin. Try not to wear cotton. It absorbs sweat and does not dry quickly. Wear socks that are synthetic like acrylic or polyester. Do not wear cotton socks. Wear running sunglasses. It helps exposure to sunlight. Apply a generous amount of sunscreen lotion before you go out in the sun.

What to Wear in Cold Weather While Running

Wear a thin synthetic fabric close to your skin. Try not to wear cotton because you end up remaining wet with sweat. As the outermost layer, wear something like nylon. It will save you from the wind. If the weather is too cold, you have to wear a layer in between. The fabric should be something thick.

Wear gloves or mittens if it is colder. Do not wear tight shoes. Wear thick socks. You can also place some disposable heat packs inside your mitten or a sock liner under your socks. You can also wear thick woolen socks.

If you wear these linings in your shoes, your shoes are bound to get tight so wear bigger sized shoes.

James Sinclair

Chapter 11
Diet and Nutrition for Runners

To maintain good health, diet is important for runners. It helps improve their performance too. Runners should make a change in their diet especially if their main aim is to lose weight. You should follow a healthy diet and avoid processed food. Have good quality meat, fruits, vegetables, nuts, seeds, and beans. Do you love junk food? It is always better to not have junk food. If you can't live without it, then once in a while is okay. If you're craving junk food, have little portions of it instead of gorging on it.

You must enjoy the food you eat. So make your healthy food appealing and interesting. Carbohydrates are good for runners but do not over eat carbohydrates. Avoid white sugar. Have a couple of vegetable servings at every meal.

Your typical breakfast could be eggs in any form with vegetables and coffee. Lunch could be a salad. Dinner could be meat with vegetables, wild rice, quinoa, zucchini noodles, brown rice, whole grain bread, etc. A little beer or wine occasionally is fine. If you can, you should sauté, bake, or grill your food instead of frying it. You can have a healthy mid-day snack in between. You can gorge on fruit when you are hungry or a handful of nuts or yogurt. An occasional helping of ice cream won't harm either.

If you want to lose weight it is better to have as few carbohydrates as possible. A Paleo diet or a Ketogenic diet or an Atkins diet will help. Do not starve yourself to lose weight. It will not help. Eat the right food.

Before your workout you can have some simple carbohydrates. Coffee before a run helps. Have it at least half an hour before a run. It will help you run faster. Sleep is also necessary so sleep well.

The main aim for losing weight in runners is to lose body fat and increase lean body mass. Excess body weight makes you lethargic and you tend to run slowly. You feel you are dragging your body. To lose body fat, have food such that your calorie intake per day is reduced. Remember, everyone's body structure is different. What works for one may not work for another.

Lean body mass can be increased by exercising and strength training. To maintain overall health and lose weight, you should first find out how many calories you need in a day. You should never have less than 1200 calories in a day. A very low calorie diet is not going to help you lose weight. Instead it will make you lethargic and you will start feeling ill. If you wish to lose one pound in a week, then reduce your calorie intake by 500 calories every day. About 50% of your calories should come from carbohydrates, 25% of your calories should be proteins, and 25% should be fats.

A Few Tips:

• Eat 5-6 smaller meals in a day instead of bigger and lesser meals. Enjoy your food.

•   Runners need carbohydrates as fuel for their body. So go in for whole grain bread and pasta. They contain more fiber and are more nutritious. Whole grains keep you with a feeling of fullness. You will feel full for a longer time. Avoid white bread or white pasta or for that matter any food items made with white flour. Quinoa is a good alternative to whole grains. Sweet potato is a good form of carbohydrates. It is an antioxidant and has vitamins, potassium and iron. Low fat yogurt has carbohydrates too. Bananas are very good for runners. It is loaded with potassium. It prevents cramps and regulates the contraction of muscle. You can have a banana as it is or make a smoothie of it.

•   Runners need proteins. Proteins are needed to build muscles. They are needed to repair the muscles. Eggs are a good source of proteins. By consuming an egg a day, you will be getting a part of your protein needs for the day. Eggs help the bones. It also helps repair muscle. Have the eggs in any form you like at any meal but it is best suited at breakfast. Beans are a good source of protein too. They have fiber as well. Meat and salmon are good sources of protein. Salmon is loaded with vitamins and minerals apart from protein. Low fat yogurt is full of proteins. You can have it as a mid-morning snack along with chopped fruits in it or churn it into a smoothie. Meat is full of proteins. Have lean cut meat and poultry. Peanut butter is very good for runners with a good amount of protein and fiber.

•   Carrots are good finger foods for runners. You can snack on it anytime. It has vitamin A that helps build a strong immune system. Low in calories, they are filling too. It is very good for losing weight. You can snack on cucumbers as they are low on calories too.

•   Look for recipes of your favorite food that can be lower in fat made with low fat ingredients. This way you can satisfy your tastes as well as maintain a healthy diet.

•   Have lots of fruits like apple, orange, peach, banana, pineapple, berries, kiwis, melons, etc. Vegetables like greens, carrots, cabbage, beans, peas, eggplant, cauliflower, broccoli, etc. Have fewer starchy vegetables and more whole grains like rice, pasta, wild rice, quinoa, oats, and couscous. It helps you feel full. You can have occasional small portions of noodles, pasta, white bread, etc. Try to eat more at breakfast, lesser at lunch, and least at dinner.

• A typical breakfast should contain proteins, low fat milk, yogurt with fruit, or a smoothie and whole wheat bread.

• You can use weight loss apps to help you track down the calories you consumed and burned.

• Do eat your favorite foods occasionally but have only small portions if they are junk foods.

• Have regular checkups with your doctor.

• Reduce the number of calories you consume.

• Gradually increase the number of calories you burn daily.

• Have proteins like lean meat, eggs, soy protein, seafood, low fat cheese, low fat hot dogs, and low fat yogurt. It is good to have a breakfast with high proteins in it.

• Have fats like all oils, avocado, nuts like almonds, cashews, walnuts, pistachios, peanut butter, almond butter, light mayonnaise, etc. Have low fat salad dressings. Avoid hydrogenated fats. Olive oil is very healthy.

• Try to have most of the carbohydrates before your run. Try to keep to the proteins and fats after the run.

• Do not stay hungry for long.

• Have lots of liquids. Water should be at the top of the list. Try and have sugarless tea. Have lots of green tea 3-4 times a day. Do not have readymade juices and drinks. They are loaded with sugar. Do not have aerated soft drinks like coke, etc.

• Do not run on an empty stomach. That is the worst thing one could do.

• As you start losing weight, you should keep adjusting your calorie intake.

• Sports drinks, energy drinks, and energy bars are good during the run as well as after the run.

James Sinclair

Chapter 12
Recipes for Homemade Energy Drinks

Energy drinks keep you hydrated and pumped while running. You can either buy them or even make them at home! Here are a few recipes to make your own energy drinks. They are easy to make and very tasty too.

1. Cranberry Sports Drink:

Ingredients:

- 1 ½ cups cranberry juice, unsweetened

- 2 ½ cups water

- ¼ teaspoon salt

- 1 tablespoon maple syrup

- ½ a star anise (optional)

Method:

1.   Add all the ingredients. Cover and keep aside for about an hour. Discard the star anise. Refrigerate and serve.

2. Strawberry Sports Drink:

Ingredients:

- 6 cups hot water

- 1 cup orange juice

- 2 lemons, juiced

- ¼ cup honey

- Stevia to taste

- ½ teaspoon salt

- 1 container strawberries, sliced

Method:

1.   Mix together all the ingredients. Let it cool naturally. Refrigerate overnight.

2.   Strain. Sip the drink and enjoy the strawberries.

3. Citrus Coconut Sports Drink:

Ingredients:

*   800 ml coconut water

*   1 teaspoon extra virgin coconut oil

*   3 teaspoons fresh lime juice

*   2 teaspoon fresh lemon juice

*   4 medjool dates, deseeded

*   3 teaspoons agave nectar

*   A large pinch sea salt

Method:

1.   Blend together all the ingredients. Chill and serve.

4. Berry Blast:

Ingredients:

*   ½ ripe banana, chopped

*   ½ cup yogurt

- ¼ cup raspberries

- ¼ cup blueberries

- ½ cup strawberries

- ¼ cup fresh orange juice

Method:

1. Blend together all the ingredients. Chill and serve.

5. Tropical Smoothie:

Ingredients:

- 1 ripe banana, chopped

- 1 peach

- 4 ounces pineapple, chopped

- ¼ cup mango, chopped

- 2 tablespoons crushed oats

Method:

1. Blend together all the ingredients. Chill and serve.

6. Chocolate Banana Smoothie:

Ingredients:

- ½ ripe banana, chopped

- 1 scoop chocolate ice cream

- 5 chocolate buttons

- ½ cup of milk

- Ice

Method:

1.   Blend together all the ingredients. Chill and serve.

7. Peanut Butter Smoothie:

Ingredients:

- 1 ripe banana, chopped

- 1 tablespoon Greek Yogurt

- 1 tablespoon peanut butter

- ½ cup milk

Method:

1.   Blend together all the ingredients. Chill and serve.

8. Homemade Protein Shake:

Ingredients:

- 2 bananas, chopped

- 1 cup low fat yogurt or soy yogurt

- 1 cup part skim milk

- 2 tablespoons peanut butter

- 2 tablespoons chia seeds

- 1 teaspoon ground cinnamon

Method:

1.   Blend together all the ingredients. Chill and serve.

9. Mango Energy Drink:

Ingredients:

- 1 cup spinach

- ½ cup frozen mango

- ¼ cup baby carrots

- ¼ cup coconut water

- ¼ cup orange juice

- 1 mandarin orange, peeled, cut into segments, deseeded

- ¼ cup yogurt

Method:

1. Blend together all the ingredients. Chill and serve.

10. **Green Smoothie:**

Ingredients:

- 3 cups spinach

- 1 ½ cups frozen peaches

- ¾ cup fresh banana, chopped

- ¾ cup raw zucchini, chopped

- 1 ¼ cup coconut water

- ¾ cup yogurt

- 3 tablespoons wheat germ

Method:

1.   Blend together all the ingredients. Chill and serve.

Chapter 13
Stay Motivated

No matter how much we want to run, staying motivated over a long period of time can be difficult. The training plan in Chapter 5 is for eight weeks. That is the equivalent of two months and two months is a long time!

There are a number of ways to stay motivated, however. Remember, you are running to improve your fitness and lose weight! Let's look at a few quick tips for staying motivated.

Set Goals

At the beginning of the training plan, set yourself a weight loss goal. Don't let it be something unobtainable. Keep it realistic and within reach. You should have a fair idea of how much weight you think you can lose over the eight weeks. When you don't feel like running, remember your goal and what you want to achieve. Keep your eye on the prize!

Get a Running Buddy

Running with someone is a great way to stay motivated. On days that you do not feel like hitting the tarmac, a running buddy is often the motivation needed to get out there and do it anyway. The great thing is that this works both ways. On some days, you may need to motivate your running buddy!

Try Different Running Routes

We all get bored with repetition, and the same goes for runners. Running the same route over and over again can become extremely boring, extremely quickly. Try a different route every week. You could even consider trading the tarmac for a nice trail run.

Consider Music

Music is often a great way to take your mind off running down miles and miles of tarmac. Load up an MP3 player with your favorite tunes and watch the miles fly by!

Treat Yourself

Another great motivator is to treat yourself for sticking to your goal. This could be something simple like a nice healthy meal at a local restaurant or even a long massage to ease those weary legs.

Consider How Lucky You Are

Many people that would like to run do not have the opportunity. Go out there and enjoy the chance you have been given.

James Sinclair

Chapter 14
Checking Your Progress

Now is the time for a reality check up. We have listed so many points here and now you need to truly determine if the points have actually brought you any significant benefits. You will have to closely observe the details.

Try and measure your weight. Did your weight decrease even a little? Even if you have not lost weight, do not be disappointed. Weight loss isn't merely determined by the number of pounds you lose. Sometimes, your body gets toned up in anticipation of weight loss and the lean body mass gets impacted. These are important parameters too.

It is a proven fact that running is bound to have a positive impact on your weight loss goal. However, like we told you before, it is not sufficient on its own. You will have to work hard to make sure that running can bring a speedy loss in weight.

So, make it a point to closely analyze the points you have implemented and the ones that you still need to work on. The points we listed in the book have been carefully compiled after observing a plethora of different factors. So, you should not rush and take your time to come up with the perfect routine that will help you get rid of all the extra weight and attain the kind of figure you will be happy to have.

If you have started experiencing the right changes, it is a healthy sign and you should continue with these tips and regime. Those who are still able to find any loss in weight should not lose hope. You can re-assess the program and then continue to work towards improvement of your body shape. Success is sure to come, sooner or later.

How Much Weight Could I lose

The amount of weight you could lose really depends on a number of different criteria. Here are the four most important.

Your Starting Weight

The weight in which you begin your program will have a huge impact on how much weight you can lose. Obviously if you are only 10 pounds overweight then you aren't going to lose much more.

If on the other hand you are 100 pounds overweight you will lose much more. There is also the fact that larger people will burn calories quicker. This is simply down to having to move their body around. The heavier you are the harder your body needs to work to move you.

You will also have a higher basal metabolic rate meaning your body will use more calories just keeping you alive. The general rule is the larger you are the more calories you will burn.

Your Sex

Your sex will also determine how many calories you can burn. Men are generally more muscular so they will usually burn more calories over the long term.

This doesn't mean that every man will burn more than every woman. If a woman works hard and has weight to lose then they can still burn more weight than men. It is just another factor to remember.

How Clean is Your Diet?

A big factor determining how much weight you can lose is how clean your diet is. This is in fact probably the biggest factor.

Your diet will determine how much weight you lose because if you get it right it will actually allow you to do more running. If you get it wrong however it will prevent you from running as effectively as you would like.

Keep your diet clean with fresh unprocessed foods as much as you can. If you want to super turbo charge your weight loss then cutting out bread (which is technically processed) will be a good way to do it.

How Hard You Work

The final factor to how much weight you can lose is down to how hard you work. Go running once a week and you will get a certain result. Go running 3 times a week and you will get a better result.

However, this can work both ways. Run too much and you can end up with exhaustion and injury that in the long term will stop you from running and stall your weight loss.

How hard you can work will be related to how clean your diet is. Keeping it low in processed food keeps your blood sugar low, this keeps insulin low which allows your body to release fat stores. With your fat releasing its energy you will have plenty available to encourage you to go running. It is for that reason that eating clean is so important.

James Sinclair

Chapter 15
Different Running Options

Running Clubs

If you want to take your running to a completely new level, then try joining a running club. Most towns have them these days. They are great for meeting other people who love running, many of whom are really good runners.

It is a great place to go to push yourself and ultimately improve your running. It will be tough but tough just means you are working hard and working hard means you are burning calories, which results in weight loss.

Many people who use running to lose weight become runners for life. It shouldn't be seen as a short term solution. It is a long term hobby and running clubs are the place many people go to keep that hobby going.

Adding a Gradient

If you add a gradient your work rate will go through the roof. This is easy to do on a treadmill as they all have a gradient setting but not so easy to do running on the street.

Most towns will have hillier areas allowing you to alter your running route to take full advantage of the gradient. If you live in a flatter area then the treadmill could be a solution for one of your runs each week.

For example, you could have a fast run, a long run and a gradient run to really mix it up.

When it comes to progression it is all about pushing your boundaries. This could be by adding a gradient, joining a club, or simply beating old personal bests. It really is up to you.

Running for Charity

As I have mentioned above, I got into charity running a few years ago and since my first run I have been obsessed. I had a couple of years out but I am back and as passionate as ever.

The great thing about running for a charity is that you can give yourself a challenge while raising money for a charity. What could be better than that?

There are loads around and they have people of all abilities. Simply go online and search for them. They are such great fun.

Challenges

Below are a number of the running challenges I did which helped keep me focused on my fitness and speed rather than just on weight loss. By working to go faster for longer you push your body. When you do that the weight loss will come as a consequence. Try them for yourself.

1 Mile Challenge

A challenge perfect for the treadmill, the 1 mile challenge is exactly what it sounds like. Your goal is to run 1 mile as fast as you can.

A mile may not seem like much but when you begin to up the speed it gets tough quickly. This is a challenge that will improve your speed to no end. It is a challenge that will push you to the limit each and every time you do it no matter how fit you get.

My advice is to not go flat out the first time. Try it and see what it is like. Use the first attempt to get a time on the board giving you something to beat. I would then keep track of my average speed so I knew next time what average speed I would need to beat. The treadmill will tell you this so remember to remember it.

The next time you get on the treadmill you will need to run faster than the previous average time to set a new personal best. After that, simply repeat and within a few weeks you will be running at a much faster pace.

WARNING: This is always a tough run because you are always aiming to run faster than ever before. Be prepared to really feel it. I love this challenge.

2 Mile Challenge

The 2 mile challenge is twice the distance of the 1 mile and should be treated in a similar way but this is tough in a completely different way.

The 1 mile challenge is all about pace and power. The 2 mile run on the other hand begins to bring in an element of stamina. For this reason, you will not be able to run at the same pace.

While it may be slower it will still test you and push you to your limits. This is a run that is all about pacing yourself for the full 3200 meters.

My advice is to set a time as with the previous challenge and to cut the time down in much the same way. I would however alternate attempts with the 1 mile and the 3 mile challenge below. This is because each challenge will help you train for the other challenges. The 1 mile challenge will help with your speed and the 3 mile will help with stamina, both of which will be needed for this challenge.

3 Mile Challenge

The 3 mile challenge is probably the longest run you will want to do on a treadmill. Anything longer and it can get really boring.

This is even more about stamina, and judging a good speed is vital to getting a good time. The important thing is to set out at a pace you can do and slowly increase it as you go.

I have put an example of what I would do when I first started running this distance. The first number is the distance travelled and the second is the speed. Therefore 400m – 10.5kph – means the first 400 meters travelled was at 10.5 kilometers per hour.

400m – 10.5kph

800m – 10.6kph

1200m – 10.7kph

1600m – 10.8kph

2000m – 10.9kph

2400m – 11.0kph

2800m – 11.1kph

3200m – 11.2kph

3600m – 11.3kph

4000m – 11.4kph

4400m – 11.5kph

4800m – 11.6kph

As the time goes by you are obviously going to get more tired, especially as the speed is increasing. The idea is that by the time you find it really hard work you are close enough to the end to keep going. The next time you can simply start on a higher number.

This will help your stamina to no end but will be run a lot slower than the 1 mile challenge.

10k Challenge

The 10kms run is probably my favorite distance because you can train for it no matter how out of shape you are but it is still a really impressive distance. If you have any level of fitness then you can train for it in just a couple of months.

So where do you begin? Well as I suggest in this book when you first start running you have no idea how far you can run. For this reason, you need to set a distance on your first run. From there you can then begin to increase it each time. The speed isn't so important at this point; you just want to get to a point where you can do the distance.

Your distances may look something like this.

First Run – 1km

Second Run – 1.8kms

Third Run – 3kms

Fourth Run – 5kms

Fifth Run – 6.7kms

Sixth Run – 8.2kms

Seventh Run – 10kms

Of course it will vary from person to person depending on everything from how much extra weight you are carrying to how competitive you are and even how much time you have free. Even the time of year could have a bearing.

The important thing is that you continue to build up the distance until you reach the 10kms mark. At this point you now know you can run the distance. It is now time to begin to work on improving your time.

A wise man once said there is only one way to train for a run and that is to run. So just keep running.

Half Marathon

This for me is where it all gets very serious. A half marathon shouldn't be attempted if you still have a large amount of weight to lose. It is a serious commitment. I would also advise you to do at least one 10km run first before moving up to the half marathon.

So how do you even begin training for a half marathon? Well there are two methods. There is the standard method where you run 3 or 4 times a week on set days running at different paces so one may be really fast, one is fast and slow, and then the long run. A typical example of this method is below.

	Mon	Tue	Wed	Thu	Fri	Sat	Sun
Week 1	Rest Day	30 minutes easy run	30 minutes easy run	Rest Day	30 minutes easy run	Rest Day	Long run: 3 miles
Week 2	Rest Day	30 minutes easy run	30 minutes tempo	Rest Day	30 minutes easy run	Rest Day	Long run: 40 minutes
Week 3	Rest Day	30 minutes easy run	40 minutes tempo	Rest Day	30 mins easy run	Rest Day	Long run: 5 miles
Week 4	Rest Day	40 minutes easy run	50 minutes tempo	Rest Day	30 mins at speed	Rest Day	Long run: 60 minutes
Week 5	Rest Day	40 minutes easy run	30 minutes tempo	Rest Day	40 mins at speed	Rest Day	Long run: 7 miles
Week 6	Rest Day	40 minutes easy run	50 minutes tempo	Rest Day	30 mins at speed	Rest Day	Long run: 8 miles
Week 7	Rest Day	40 minutes easy	40 minutes tempo	Rest Day	40 mins at speed	Rest Day	Long run: 60 minutes

		run					
Week 8	Rest Day	40 minutes easy run	40 minutes tempo	Rest Day	40 mins at speed	Rest Day	Long run: 10 miles
Week 9	Rest Day	40 minutes easy run	50 minutes tempo	Rest Day	50 mins at speed	Rest Day	Long run: 5 miles
Week 10	Rest Day	40 minutes easy run	40 minutes tempo	Rest Day	40 mins at speed	Rest Day	Long run: 12 miles
Week 11	Rest Day	40 minutes easy run	40 minutes tempo	Rest Day	40 mins at speed	Rest Day	Long run: 6 miles
Week 12	Rest Day	40 minutes easy run	40 minutes tempo	Rest Day	50 mins easy run	Rest Day	Half marathon race

This does take a lot of your time and in all honesty I am not a believer that you need to do that much running. I think 2 runs a week is plenty if you give yourself enough time to train. One run should be fast and one should be long.

Keep the fast one to a shorter distance as you won't be able to run so far if you are running at pace. The real work though is done on the long run. For this you will need to increase it from whatever you can already do up to the half marathon distance.

So if you can already do a 10km run before you start training you could increase it by 1km each week through your long run so it would look something like this:

Week 1 – 10kms

Week 2 – 11kms

Week 3 – 12kms

Week 4 – 13kms

Week 5 – 14kms

Week 6 – 15kms

Week 7 – 16kms

Week 8 – 17kms

Week 9 – 18kms

Week 10 – 19kms

Week 11 – 20kms

Week 12 – 21kms

Once you have run the full distance you will know in your mind that it is achievable. With this belief comes a lot more confidence and with that you can kick on to working on improving your time.

By the time race day arrives you will have done the run a few times and be ultra confident that you will be able to do yourself justice.

Note: The last couple of weeks before the run slowly reduce the amount of running you do. This is called tapering and it is a strategy to make sure you are fit and ready to do the main event.

Full Marathon

For many the marathon is the pinnacle of physical challenges. A marathon is 26.2 miles or just over 42 kilometers. It is a tough race that any participant should take very seriously. It will take some dedicated training over a number of months. Unlike a 5km fun run this is an event that you simply must train for.

Due to the distance and the strain it puts on the body the training alone is too much for many people with injuries picked up before the event being common place. That just goes to show just how tough the event is.

The marathon is in reality only to be considered once you have completed a half marathon. Only then can you really get any sort of idea how tough it can be having proved you are up for the serious training. Even after a half marathon it is hard to understand just how tough the full one can be.

My advice for running a marathon is training, training, and more training.

Training Basics

As with all running, but particularly when running such distances, it is important to remember that there is more to running a marathon than just running. You must also remember the warm up and cool down. You need to do this with all running but particularly with the marathon.

The warm up is ideally going to be a less intense version of what you will be doing. You could start with a walk or light jog. DO NOT stretch before you warm up. This is a sure fire way to pull a muscle. Once you have warmed up for 5 – 10 minutes you can have a light stretch although it is not essential.

Once you have done your run you will need to cool off. This will be similar to the warm up. Slow down and run or walk at a greatly reduced pace allowing your muscles to cool down gradually. Once you have cooled down and you are getting your breath back you will need to stretch.

While stretching wasn't so important in your warm up it is vital in the cool down. Ensure that you stretch all of your muscles to prevent your body from becoming tight and out of alignment.

My Marathon Training Technique

The hardest thing about training for a marathon is simply the distance. It is highly likely that on your first attempt you will be happy with just completing the course so a time is not so important. This is good as it allows you to focus purely on being physically able to do the 26.2 miles.

Now I am assuming here that you have done at least a 10km run before and hopefully for your sake quite regularly. If not, then I would suggest working towards a 10km run first.

So you can do a 10km. The next step is to begin to step up your distance. Remember that time doesn't matter too much on your first marathon. Just prove that you can do the distance and worry about a time on your second run.

So How Do You Up The Distance?

Simply by running is the short answer. If you can do 10km then begin to build it up between 1km and 2km each long run. You should try and do a long run once a week so your body has time to repair and improve in between. I would also do a mid-week short fast run but that is totally up to you.

Your weekly targets could be something like this:

Week 1 – 12kms

Week 2 – 14kms

Week 3 – 16kms

Week 4 – 18kms

Week 5 – 20kms

Week 6 – 22kms

Week 7 – 24kms

Week 8 – 26kms

Week 9 – 28kms

Week 10 – 30kms

Week 11 – 32kms

Week 12 – 34kms

Week 13 – 36kms

Week 14 – 38kms

Week 15 – 40kms

Week 16 – 42kms

It is totally up to you as to whether you train right up to the full distance. There is something nice about standing on the start line knowing you can and already have done the distance.

You can also slow your training down a little increasing by 1km each week. This will take you twice as long but with smaller increases your body should be able to cope with that level of improvement quite comfortably.

If you can already run a half marathon then simply start your long run from 21kms rather than 10km. This will slow down the time it will take you to train.

Many marathon training plans suggest running up to 4 times a week. I believe with proper nutrition, good quality warm ups, warm downs, stretches, and a decent long run you won't need to run that often. Twice a week is fine if you make one run short and fast and one you make as your long run.

Now it is simply down to you running until you can run a marathon distance. Remember to give yourself plenty of training time and more than anything else, respect the distance.

Chapter 16
Other Options to Consider

There are a number of other aspects connected to running that you will need to consider each time you step outside your door in your running shoes.

Keep Hydrated

As you run, you begin to sweat. This expels important fluids out of your body, and it is essential that you replace these liquids. Let's take a look at a few tips for keeping hydrated while you run.

Drink Water along Your Route

Either take water with you while you run or stop and drink water along the way. For every 20 minutes that you run try to drink around 200 to 300 milliliters of water. If you are running for a long period, you might consider a sports drink to help replace any electrolytes your body has lost. A word of warning, you can overhydrate. Listen to your body, muscles consist mostly of water. If you suddenly feel fatigued, the chances are your body needs water.

Consider Fruits

A fruit is a great way to get some fluids into your body as well as important vitamins, minerals, and electrolytes. Bananas, which are high in potassium, are a great fruit to eat while you run. Do not let a fruit replace water, however; you will still need to drink regularly.

Weigh Yourself Before and After

Weigh yourself before you begin your run and again straight after. If your weight drops by 3%, you might be dehydrated. Replacing water lost through exercise is just as important in the hours after the exercise is finished.

Pay Attention to Your Mouth

Dehydration often manifests itself in the form of a dry mouth. If your mouth starts to get dry or parched, drink water immediately.

Check Your Skin

Another way to see if you are keeping your body hydrated is to pinch the fleshy skin near the back of your hand. If it returns into position fairly quickly your hydration levels are fine. If it takes some time, you might be starting to become dehydrated. Stop and drink some water!

Running Indoors

You might be lucky enough to either own a treadmill or have a gym membership and, therefore, have access to a treadmill.

Treadmills are a great way to continue your running plan, especially if the weather takes a turn for the worse. Running on a treadmill is very different to running on the open road, however. These handy tips can help you prepare for a run indoors.

Be Prepared

This would appear to be pretty obvious, but once you have started on a treadmill you do not want to get off until your run is over. Make sure you have everything with you that you might need including water and a towel to wipe down, especially if you do not own the treadmill!

Equipment wise, running on a treadmill is no different to running outside. Ensure you have the correct running clothes, socks, and of course, your running shoes.

Don't Forget to Warm Up

Again, warming up correctly is just as important before a session on the treadmill as it is when running on the road. Perform your pre-run stretches and once you begin on the treadmill itself, start off slowly. Follow this great treadmill warm up - walk for 3 minutes, jog for 3 minutes, and then ease into a run, increasing the speed slowly until you reach a comfortable level.

Use the Incline

One advantage of a treadmill is that it can simulate hills whenever you want; great for the incline running section of our training plan in Chapter 5. Running up an incline is also an excellent way to get your heart rate up and to burn more calories!

Don't Forget to Warm Down

A proper warm down is just as important as your warm up. Many people use this simple equation to warm down after a treadmill run. Walk on the treadmill for 1 minute for every mile you have covered during your run. Don't forget to stretch afterward.

James Sinclair

Conclusion

Thank you for purchasing this book. I hope you found the tips and guidelines mentioned in this book helpful. Running is indeed a pleasurable and healthy way to reduce weight if done in the right manner.

There are many ways to lose weight but running is one of the easiest and healthiest ways. If you have the willpower to follow through with the activity and if you follow the diet properly, you will definitely see a change in you and your body.

Once you are able to overcome the initial running phase, you will find the feeling and euphoria of running addictive. It is just the matter of perseverance. So get your running shoes out and get running.

Thank you once again and keep running!

James Sinclair

www.ingramcontent.com/pod-product-compliance
Lightning Source LLC
Chambersburg PA
CBHW060521290526
45791CB00001B/482